BREAST CANCER

A Comprehensive Guide on All you
Need to Know about Breast Cancer

Dr. JANE ROCK

Table of Contents

CHAPTER ONE

Introduction

Breast cancer is a common and often life-changing health condition that affects people all over the world, regardless of age, gender, or culture. The purpose of this comprehensive reference is to give a foundation for understanding breast cancer by covering three major aspects: an overview of breast cancer, the importance of breast health, and the purpose of this comprehensive guide.

Overview of Breast Cancer.

Breast cancer develops in the cells of the breast. It affects both men and women, however it is more typically diagnosed in women. The disease can take several forms, the most prevalent being invasive ductal carcinoma. Breast cancer can also arise in other areas of the breast, such as the ducts, lobules, or connective tissue.

Understanding breast cancer requires recognizing aberrant cell proliferation, which can lead to tumor formation. These tumors might be benign (not cancerous) or malignant (cancerous). Malignant tumors can infect neighboring tissues and, in some situations, spread to other parts of the body via the bloodstream or lymphatic system.

Understanding the many forms, phases, and characteristics of breast cancer is critical for making educated decisions and implementing appropriate management. This guide will delve into the complexities of breast cancer, providing insights to provide readers with the information they require.

Importance of Breast Health

Breast health is an essential component of overall well-being, and addressing it is critical in the early identification and prevention of breast cancer. Regular breast self-exams, clinical breast examinations, and mammography screenings all help to detect changes in breast tissue in a timely manner.

Understanding and actively supporting breast health is important not only for women, but also for men, because breast cancer can impact people of any gender. Early detection enhances the likelihood of successful therapy and better outcomes. As a result, raising awareness about breast health is a preventative step that has the potential to save lives.

Purpose of this Guide

The goal of this book is to provide individuals with information about breast cancer, from the basics to the most recent advances in research and treatment. This handbook is a comprehensive resource for anyone who has been directly affected by breast cancer, a caregiver, or someone who is interested in prevention.

The handbook tries to:

• Educate on breast cancer, including causes, risk factors, and kinds.

• Empower readers with information about early detection,

screening protocols, and sustaining breast health.

• Support: Offer insights into the emotional and psychological elements of dealing with breast cancer, along with resources for support and coping methods.

• Provide an update on recent breast cancer research and treatment options.

• Guide: Offer practical counsel to people receiving treatment, living with breast cancer, or adjusting to life after treatment.

This guide intends to be a beneficial companion on the journey toward better breast health and overall well-being by providing a holistic approach to breast cancer awareness, prevention, and management.

Understanding the Anatomy of the Breast

Structure and Function of the Breast

The human breast is a complicated and convoluted organ made up mostly of glandular tissue, ducts, fatty tissue, and connective tissue. Its principal role is to create milk for breastfeeding, so assisting in the nutrition of neonates. The following are the important components:

• **Glandular Tissue:** The part of the breast that produces milk. It is made up of lobes, which are further divided into smaller lobules. Each lobule contains clusters of alveoli, which are small sacs that generate milk.

Ducts are slender tubes that transport milk from the lobules to the nipple. When a mother is lactating, her milk flows through these ducts to the baby during breastfeeding.

• The breast's connective tissue provides structural stability. This tissue serves to keep the breast's form and location stable.

• The breast contains adipose tissue, which contributes to its shape and size. The distribution of fat differs between individuals, influencing breast appearance.

Understanding the structure of the breast is critical for understanding breast health since different types of cells and tissues can cause a variety of illnesses, including breast cancer.

Types of Breast Tissue

Breast tissues are usually classified into two types: glandular (epithelial) tissue and stromal (connective and fatty).

• Glandular Tissue: Contains the lobes and lobules responsible for milk production. It is made up of epithelial cells and is essential for nursing.

• Connective tissue refers to the fibrous and fatty tissue that surrounds and supports glandular tissue. Connective tissue aids in the preservation of the breast's structure and integrity.

Understanding the distribution and balance of these tissues is critical for interpreting breast imaging, such as mammograms, and identifying abnormalities.

Hormonal influences

Hormones have an important role in the growth and function of the breast. The key hormones involved are estrogen and progesterone, both generated by the ovaries. These hormones have an impact on several areas of breast health, including:

•   Puberty: Hormonal changes during puberty accelerate the development of the mammary glands and ducts, resulting in breast expansion.

•   Menstrual Cycle: Hormonal fluctuations might affect breast tissue density and sensitivity.

•   During pregnancy, hormonal changes prepare the breasts for milk production, resulting in the formation of glandular tissue.

• Menopause: As women approach menopause, hormonal changes cause a decrease in breast density as well as changes in breast composition.

Understanding hormonal impacts allows us to appreciate the dynamic nature of breast health throughout a woman's life, as well as gain insight into the elements that influence breast cancer risk and development. This knowledge is critical for both preserving breast health and evaluating changes that occur over time.

Breast Cancer Definitions and Types

Breast cancer is a complex disease that occurs when abnormal cells in the breast grow uncontrollably. Understanding the core ideas of breast cancer, including its definition and numerous kinds, is critical for raising awareness and education.

Definition of breast cancer:

Breast cancer is a tumor that begins in the cells of the breast. The breast is made up of several tissues, including glandular tissues that generate milk, ducts that carry milk, fatty and connective tissues that provide structure, and lymphatic tissues that participate in the immune system.

When normal cells in the breast receive genetic changes, they can become cancer cells. These cancer cells can form a mass or lump known as a tumor, which has the potential to infect nearby tissues or spread to other parts of the body.

It is crucial to understand that not all breast tumors are malignant. Some tumors are benign (non-cancerous) and pose no risk to health, but others are malignant (cancerous) and require immediate care and treatment.

Breast Cancer Types:

Breast cancer is a complex illness with various subtypes, each defined by the individual cells involved and their characteristics. Here are a few common types:

• DCIS (Ductal Carcinoma In Situ) is a non-invasive breast cancer where abnormal cells are identified in the duct lining but have not spread to surrounding tissues. It is frequently regarded as a precancerous stage.

• The most prevalent type of breast cancer is invasive ductal carcinoma (IDC), which begins in the milk ducts and spreads to adjacent breast tissues. It can also spread to other areas of the body.

• Invasive Lobular Carcinoma (ILC): This type of cancer starts in the lobules (milk-producing glands) and spreads to adjacent tissues. While less prevalent than IDC, ILC is more difficult to identify using imaging.

• Triple-Negative Breast Cancer: This subtype lacks estrogen and progesterone receptors, as well as the HER2 protein. It could be more aggressive and resistant to some therapies.

• HER2-Positive Breast Cancer: Overexpression of the HER2 protein promotes cancer cell proliferation. Targeted treatments such as Herceptin are frequently utilized in treatment.

•	Hormone Receptor-Positive Breast Cancer: Cancers that have estrogen and/or progesterone receptors fall under this category. These receptors influence cancer growth and are targeted in hormone therapy.

Causes and Risk Factors of Breast Cancer

Understanding the causes and risk factors of breast cancer is critical to both prevention and early detection. While the specific etiology of breast cancer is not always known, many risk factors have been identified.

Causes of breast cancer:

Breast cancer is caused by a complex combination of genetic, hormonal, environmental, and lifestyle factors. While it is not always possible to pinpoint a single cause, scientists have found various significant factors:

• Certain genes, such BRCA1 and BRCA2, have inherited mutations that raise the risk of getting breast cancer. However, the majority of breast cancers are not directly caused by inherited gene abnormalities.

• Hormonal Influences: Hormones such as estrogen and progesterone can influence breast cell proliferation. Long-term exposure to these hormones, whether naturally occurring or via hormone replacement therapy

(HRT), may raise the risk of breast cancer.

• Women are more likely than males to develop breast cancer as they age. However, breast cancer can affect people of any age or gender.

• A family history of breast or ovarian cancer can increase the risk, particularly if close relatives like a mother, sister, or daughter have had the disease.

Individuals who have previously been diagnosed with breast cancer or certain non-cancerous breast disorders may be at a higher risk.

Breast Cancer Risk Factors:

Several risk factors can increase the likelihood of acquiring breast cancer. It's important to emphasize that having one or more risk factors doesn't guarantee you'll get breast cancer, and many people who get the disease have no recognized risks. The following are examples of common risk factors:

• Gender and age: Being a woman and aging are two major risk factors. Women are at a larger risk than men, and this risk rises with age.

• Family History: Having a first-degree family (mother, sister, or daughter) with breast cancer raises the risk, especially if diagnosed at a young age.

• Certain inherited gene mutations, including BRCA1 and BRCA2, can dramatically raise the risk of breast cancer.

• Certain reproductive factors, such as early menstruation, late menopause, having a child after 30, or not having children, can increase the chance of developing breast cancer.

• Long-term use of hormone replacement therapy (HRT), especially a combination of estrogen and progesterone, may raise risk.

• Previous chest radiation therapy for other cancers, particularly during adolescence, increases the risk.

• Women with thick breast tissue may be more likely to get breast cancer.

Common Signs and Symptoms:

Identifying the signs and symptoms of breast cancer is critical for early detection. While the appearance of these symptoms does not always imply breast cancer, they should warrant further evaluation by a healthcare expert.

1. The most typical sign is the appearance of a painless lump or tumor in the breast or underarm.

2. Breast Appearance Changes: Changes in the size, shape, or appearance of the breast.

3. Skin changes include redness, dimpling, or puckering on the breast.

4. Nipple alterations include inversion, drainage, and skin changes.

5. Pain: Although breast cancer is not always painful, some people may feel discomfort or pain.

CHAPTER TWO

Screening and Early Detection

Understanding the importance of early detection is critical for improving overall breast health and outcomes in breast cancer. Early detection entails detecting the presence of cancer in its early stages, frequently before any symptoms develop. Breast self-exams are one of the most important strategies for early detection.

The importance of early detection:

• Improved Treatment alternatives: Early identification of breast cancer provides more treatment alternatives. When cancer is detected early, it is frequently localized, making it more curable and increasing the likelihood of a happy outcome.

• Early detection of breast cancer leads to increased survival rates. The earlier cancer is detected, the more likely it will be successfully treated, resulting in higher long-term survival.

• Early-stage breast cancer may require fewer aggressive treatments than advanced stages. This may have a smaller impact on general health and well-being, lowering the physical and emotional load of treatment.

• Early identification can lead to less invasive surgical procedures and preserve more natural breast tissue. This is particularly significant for women who are concerned about the cosmetic and psychological consequences of breast cancer therapy.

Breast self-examinations:

Breast self-exams are a simple and convenient way for women to monitor changes in their breasts. While not a replacement for routine professional tests and mammograms, self-exams allow people to take an active role in their breast health. Here's a beginner's guide to breast self-examinations:

When to do a breast self-exam:

•   For menstruation women, perform the test a few days after your period has ended.

•   For post-menopausal women, choose a set day each month.

Visual inspection:

• Examine your breasts in a mirror for any changes in size, shape, or symmetry.

• Check for skin changes like redness or dimpling.

• Check for nipple changes, such as inversion or discharge.

Manual Examination:

• Explore your breasts with your fingertips while lying down.

• Apply a circular motion with your fingers to cover the entire breast and underarm area.

• Keep an eye out for any lumps, thickening, or texture changes.

Consistency and regularity:

• Conduct self-exams monthly, preferably on the same day.

• Take note of any changes and notify a healthcare practitioner as soon as possible.

While breast self-exams are a useful practice, it is important to note that they are not a stand-alone tool for detecting breast cancer. A thorough screening strategy also includes regular clinical breast exams by healthcare experts and mammography.

Mammography and Other Screening Methods:

Breast cancer screening uses a variety of ways to detect abnormalities in the early stages. Mammograms are an important tool in breast cancer screening, and understanding their significance, along with other screening tools, is critical for breast health maintenance.

1. Mammograms:

• Definition: A mammogram is a low-dose X-ray imaging of the breast. It is the primary breast cancer screening tool, used to detect anomalies such as tumors or masses that cannot be palpated during a physical examination.

• Frequency: Mammograms are commonly advised once a year for women beginning around the age of 40, while individual recommendations may vary depending on factors such as family history and personal health.

• A mammography involves compressing each breast between two plates and taking X-rays from various angles. Compression is required to obtain crisp images while minimizing radiation exposure.

• The norm for mammography is digital mammography, which provides detailed images with greater visibility.

• 3D Mammography (Tomosynthesis): This technology captures numerous images from various angles to provide a more detailed and precise view, particularly in thick breast tissue.

2. Other Screening Methods:

Breast ultrasound:

• Purpose: Used to assess anomalies in mammography or for those with thick breast tissue.

• Procedure: Image of the breast is created utilizing sound waves. It's a non-invasive method that doesn't require radiation.

Breast MRI (Magnetic Resonance Imaging):

• Used for high-risk people or to evaluate aberrant mammography findings.

• Method: Magnetic fields and radio waves are used to obtain detailed pictures of the breast. This is a non-invasive treatment.

Molecular breast imaging:

• Purpose: Used when other imaging technologies do not yield clear results.

• The procedure involves injecting a small amount of radioactive material into the bloodstream, which is subsequently detected using a specific camera.

Understanding breast biopsies

If an anomaly is discovered during screening, a biopsy may be ordered to evaluate whether it is malignant. A biopsy is the removal of a tiny tissue sample for examination under a microscope.

Types of biopsies:

• Core Needle Biopsy involves removing tiny tissue samples with a hollow needle.

• Fine-Needle Aspiration (FNA) involves using a thin, hollow needle to remove fluid and cells from a lump.

• Vacuum-Assisted Biopsy: A probe collects several tissue

samples with a single needle insertion.

• Surgical biopsy: Surgical biopsy involves removing a greater amount of the abnormal tissue or the entire lump.

• Local anesthetic is commonly used for biopsies to reduce discomfort.

• Pathology examination: A pathologist examines tissue samples under a microscope to detect cancer cells and identify their type and characteristics.

Understanding the biopsy results is critical for making an accurate diagnosis and developing an effective treatment plan. Biopsies are frequently the final step in establishing whether a suspected discovery is malignant or benign.

Diagnosis and staging of breast cancer:

Navigating the diagnosis and staging procedure is critical for understanding the scope and features of breast cancer. It is critical for beginners to understand the diagnostic processes, the phases of breast cancer, and the ideas of grading and prognosis.

Procedures for Diagnosis:

Clinical Breast Examination (CBE):

• Function: A physical exam performed by a healthcare expert to detect lumps, changes in breast size or shape, or other abnormalities.

Imaging studies:

• Mammography: X-ray scans of the breast can uncover abnormalities, particularly those that are not palpable.

• Ultrasound imaging is used to detect abnormalities in mammograms.

• Magnetic Resonance Imaging (MRI) is a detailed imaging technique that uses magnetic fields and radio waves to assess high-risk individuals or specific scenarios.

Biopsy:

• Purpose: Determine if a suspicious finding is malignant or benign.

• Types include core needle biopsy, fine-needle aspiration, vacuum-assisted biopsy, and surgical biopsy.

- Procedure: A pathologist removes a tiny tissue sample for evaluation under a microscope.

Stages of breast cancer:

Breast cancer staging determines the amount and spread of malignancy. The TNM technique is extensively used to assess tumor size, lymph node involvement, and metastasis (spread). The stages are categorized from zero to four:

- **Stage 0 (In Situ):** Cancer is confined to the original spot and does not spread to neighboring tissues.

- **Stages I and II:** Localized cancer, with Stage II suggesting higher tumor size or lymph node involvement.

• **Stage III**: Cancer has spread to lymph nodes or tissues near the breast.

• **Stage IV (Metastatic):** Cancer has spread to distant organs or tissues, including the lungs, liver, bones, and brain.

Grading and prognosis:

Grades:

• Goal: To evaluate how aberrant cancer cells appear under a microscope, suggesting how quickly the cancer may spread.

• Grade 1 (Well-Differentiated): Cells resemble normal cells and grow slowly.

• Grade 2 (Moderately Differentiated): Cells exhibit abnormalities, indicating a moderate growth rate.

• Grade 3 (Poorly Differentiated): Cells appear significantly different from normal cells, indicating rapid growth.

The prognosis:

• Purpose: To anticipate illness progression and outcomes.

• Considered factors include stage, grade, hormone receptor status, HER2 status, age, overall health, and therapy response.

• Early stage, well-differentiated cancers with hormone receptor-positive and HER2-negative status are favorable prognostic indicators.

Understanding the stage, grade, and prognosis can assist guide treatment options and provide useful information about the disease's probable consequences.

Breast Cancer Treatment Options:

Navigating the numerous therapy choices for breast cancer is an important part of treating the disease properly. For those new to the field, here's an overview of three main treatment options: surgery, radiation therapy, and chemotherapy.

1. Surgery:

• Purpose: Surgery is often the first step in treating breast cancer, removing the tumor and surrounding tissues.

• Types of surgical procedures:

• Lumpectomy (Breast-Conserving Surgery): Removes the tumor as well as a small margin of healthy tissue around it. It seeks to preserve as much of the breast as feasible.

• Mastectomy: The entire breast is removed. Different types include:

i. A simple mastectomy is the removal of the entire breast.

ii. Modified Radical Mastectomy removes breast tissue and several lymph nodes.

iii. Radical mastectomy involves removing the breast, underlying chest muscles, and lymph nodes. Nowadays, it is rarely performed unless absolutely essential.

• Lymph node dissection may involve removing surrounding lymph nodes to assess cancer spread.

• Breast Reconstruction: After mastectomy, reconstructive surgery can restore the breast's look.

2. Radiation Therapy:

• Radiation therapy targets and kills cancer cells or inhibits their division and growth.

• Methodology:

• External Beam Radiation involves the patient lying on a treatment table while a machine delivers targeted radiation from outside the body.

• Internal Radiation (Brachytherapy): Radioactive sources are inserted into or close to the tumor.

• Radiation therapy can be administered after surgery

(adjuvant) to destroy cancer cells or before surgery (neoadjuvant) to reduce tumor size.

• Common side effects include weariness, skin changes, and local discomfort.

3. Chemotherapy:

• Goal: Chemotherapy is the use of medications to either kill or delay the growth of cancer cells.

• Administrative:

• Intravenous (IV): Medication is administered via a vein.

• Certain chemotherapy medications are given orally.

• Chemotherapy can be administered before surgery to decrease tumors, after surgery to target leftover cancer cells, or as the primary treatment for advanced stages.

• Common adverse effects include nausea, exhaustion, hair loss, and an elevated risk of infection. These adverse effects are being managed more effectively thanks to advances in supportive care.

4. Hormonal Therapy:

• Hormone therapy targets and blocks estrogen and progesterone, which certain breast tumors utilize to grow.

• Significance:

• Used for hormone receptor-positive breast tumors that express estrogen and/or progesterone receptors.

• Adjuvant therapy is commonly used to lower the chance of cancer recurrence following surgery.

5. Typical Medications:

• Tamoxifen is an estrogen receptor blocker used to treat both premenopausal and postmenopausal women.

• Aromatase inhibitors, such as Anastrozole, Letrozole, and Exemestane, can suppress estrogen production in postmenopausal women.

• Possible side effects include hot flashes, joint pain, and increased risk of osteoporosis.

6. Targeted therapies:

• Goal: Targeted medicines target specific molecules involved in cancer growth, allowing for a more precise and successful therapeutic approach.

• Significance:

• Used for HER2-positive breast cancer, when cells overexpress the HER2 protein.

• Used in conjunction with chemotherapy or as a single treatment.

• Typical Medications:

• Trastuzumab (Herceptin): inhibits the development of HER2-positive breast cancer cells.

• Pertuzumab: Used in conjunction with trastuzumab to improve efficacy.

• Side effects may include infusion responses, heart troubles, and, in rare circumstances, lung problems.

7. Immunotherapy:

• Immunotherapy enhances the immune system's ability to recognize and fight cancer cells.

• Significance:

• Conducting continuing research to determine optimal treatments for breast cancer.

• Used in clinical studies or in select circumstances where other treatments were unsuccessful.

• Typical Medications:

• Immune checkpoint inhibitors (Pembrolizumab, Atezolizumab) target specific proteins on cancer cells.

• Immunotherapy may produce immune-related adverse effects, including fatigue, rash, and inflammation in different organs. These are normally handled with close monitoring and, when needed, therapeutic adjustments.

CHAPTER THREE

Prevention and Risk Reduction for Breast Cancer

Taking proactive actions to prevent and minimize the risk of breast cancer entails addressing lifestyle factors, including genetic counseling and testing, and implementing preventative measures. Here's a thorough exploration for beginners:

1. Lifestyle factors:

❖ Healthy Diet:

A well-balanced diet with fruits, vegetables, whole grains, and lean proteins promotes general health. According to several research, eating a lot of fruits and vegetables may reduce your risk of developing breast cancer.

• Limit consumption of processed meals, red meat, and sugary drinks.

• The Mediterranean diet has potential health benefits.

❖ **Physical Activity on a Regular Basis:**

• Encourage regular physical activity, aiming for at least 150 minutes of moderate-intensity exercise per week.

• Include exercises like walking, running, swimming, and strength training.

❖ **Maintain a healthy weight.**

• Aim for a BMI within the suggested range.

- For effective weight management, maintain a balanced diet and exercise routine.

❖ Limit alcohol consumption.

- Limit alcohol consumption to moderate levels (one drink per day for women).

- Excessive alcohol drinking increases the risk of breast cancer.

❖ Avoid tobacco products.

- Stop smoking and reduce exposure to secondhand smoke.

- Smoking has been associated with an increased risk of acquiring breast cancer.

❖ Breastfeeding:

- Breastfeeding may protect women against breast cancer.

2. Genetic counseling and testing:

> Identifying High-Risk Individuals:

• Genetic counseling is indicated for those with a family history of breast cancer or other risk factors.

• Genetic testing may uncover mutations in genes like BRCA1 and BRCA2.

> Understanding genetic risk:

• Positive genetic tests suggest a higher risk of developing breast cancer.

• Genetic counselors offer guidance on risk management and prevention strategies.

3. Preventive Measures:

❖ Chemo-prevention:

• Women at high risk may benefit from drugs like tamoxifen or aromatase inhibitors.

• Consult a healthcare physician about the potential advantages and hazards.

❖ Prophylactic surgery.

• High-risk patients may opt for preventive mastectomy (removal of one or both breasts) or prophylactic oophorectomy.

• Surgical procedures are usually evaluated and discussed with healthcare specialists.

❖ Ongoing Screening:

• Schedule frequent breast cancer screenings, such as mammography and clinical exams.

- Early detection through screening can lead to better outcomes.

❖ Self-examinations:

- Conduct regular breast self-exams to understand the natural appearance and feel of the breasts.

- Promptly report any changes or irregularities to your healthcare physician.

❖ Hormonal Replacement Therapy (HRT):

- Consider the risks and advantages of hormone replacement treatment with a healthcare physician, particularly for postmenopausal women.

- Prolonged usage of some hormones may increase the risk of breast cancer.

Living with Breast Cancer

Receiving a breast cancer diagnosis can be a difficult and life-changing experience. It is critical to address the emotional, psychological, and practical elements of living with breast cancer. A thorough guide for beginners on coping with the diagnosis, managing mental well-being, developing support systems, and adopting lifestyle adjustments is available here.

Coping With Diagnosis:

• Understanding emotions:

Allow yourself to experience various emotions, such as fear, sadness, rage, and perplexity. It is natural to feel a range of emotions after receiving a cancer diagnosis.

• Gathering information:

Obtain accurate information on your diagnosis, treatment options, and potential adverse effects. Knowledge can help you make informed decisions and reduce worry.

• Communication with the healthcare team:

Ensure open contact with your healthcare staff. Ask questions, seek clarity, and actively engage in treatment plan decision-making.

• Obtaining Second Opinions:

Get a second opinion if necessary. Different points of view can provide new insights and assist you in making better informed decisions regarding your treatment.

Emotional and psychological dimensions:

- **Emotional Assistance:**

Speak with friends, relatives, or a therapist to express your emotions. Emotional support is critical at this difficult time and can help reduce feelings of loneliness.

- **Joining support groups:**

Join support groups for those with breast cancer. Sharing experiences with someone who understand your journey can be quite reassuring.

- **Counseling and therapy:**

Professional counseling or therapy can offer a safe environment to deal with the emotional effect of breast cancer diagnosis. Therapists can provide coping strategies and emotional support.

• Mindfulness and relaxation techniques:

Mindfulness, meditation, and deep breathing techniques can reduce stress and improve emotional well-being.

Support Systems and Resources:

• Family and friends:

Include loved ones in your trip. Their involvement can bring practical help, emotional consolation, and a sense of shared duty.

• Social Workers & Patient Navigators:

Social workers and patient navigators can help navigate the healthcare system, access resources, and offer personalized assistance.

• Cancer organizations:

Use materials offered by recognized cancer groups. These organizations frequently provide educational materials, support services, and community programming to those afflicted by breast cancer.

• Financial and legal assistance:

Inquire about potential financial and legal aid. Some groups provide assistance with medical bills, and legal specialists can advise on pertinent matters.

Lifestyle Changes:

• Nutritional Health:

A balanced and nutritious diet helps improve overall health. For personalized guidance, speak with a healthcare practitioner or a nutritionist.

• Regular exercise:

Engage in regular physical activity since it can improve mood, energy levels, and general physical health. Before beginning a new workout plan, consult with your healthcare team.

• Prioritize self-care.

Prioritize self-care activities that provide joy and relaxation. This could involve hobbies, spending time outside, or participating in creative activities.

• Balancing Work and Therapy:

If you are employed, discuss your circumstances with your employer. Discuss how you may adapt your work schedule or workload to accommodate treatment and rehabilitation.

Living with breast cancer is a challenging journey that requires physical, emotional, and lifestyle changes. Creating a solid support network, remaining informed, and addressing mental well-being can all lead to a more resilient and powerful experience. Remember that each person's path is unique, and it's fine to seek assistance and tailor your approach to your specific requirements and preferences.

Survivorship and Beyond

Navigating Life Following Breast Cancer Treatment

Completing breast cancer treatment signifies the start of a new phase of the journey: survivorship. This period is spent adjusting to life after treatment, managing follow-up care, addressing potential long-term effects, and dealing with the dread of recurrence. Here's a beginners' introduction to survivorship and what happens after.

Life after Treatment:

• Emotional transition:

Graduating from treatment might provide emotions like relief, excitement, and thankfulness. However, it is natural to feel a range of emotions while you adjust to your "new normal."

• Physical recovery:

Allow time for physical rehabilitation. Fatigue and other treatment-related side effects may remain, but your energy levels should eventually return.

• Rebuilding and Rediscovery:

Utilize this opportunity to rediscover and rebuild elements of your life. Reconnect with the hobbies, relationships, and activities that make you happy and fulfilled.

Follow-up Care:

• Regular check-ups.

Schedule follow-up appointments with your healthcare team. These check-ups usually include physical exams, imaging studies, and talks about any concerns or symptoms.

• Monitoring for recurrence.

Regular follow-up care monitors for recurrence and prompts intervention as needed. It's a vital component of maintaining breast health.

•   Communication with the healthcare team:

Ensure open contact with your healthcare staff. Discuss any persistent symptoms, concerns, or questions you have regarding your health.

Managing Long-term Effects:

•   Addressing treatment side effects.

Some survivors may endure long-term repercussions of treatment, including weariness, joint discomfort, and cognitive function abnormalities. Communicate these difficulties to your healthcare team so that they can be addressed appropriately.

•   Rehabilitation & Support Services:

Consider rehabilitation programs, such physical therapy or counseling, to address ongoing physical or emotional issues.

• Wellness Practices:

Wellness activities such as regular exercise, a good diet, and stress management can improve overall health and recovery.

Fear of recurrence

• Normalizing emotions.

Survivors often worry about recurrence. Recognize and normalize your feelings. It's acceptable to be concerned about the risk of cancer returning.

• Open Discussion:

Share your anxieties with your healthcare team. They can offer knowledge, reassurance, and support as you navigate this area of survivorship.

• Mindfulness and coping strategies:

Use mindfulness practices and coping methods to manage anxiety. Meditation, deep breathing, and connecting with support networks are all effective techniques.

• Support groups:

Think about joining a survivor support group. Sharing your issues with someone who understand them might bring you comfort and perspective.

Taking the Next Step:

Survivorship is a continuous process of adjusting and adapting. It entails accepting a new sense of normalcy, regulating bodily and mental well-being, and remaining watchful for follow-up treatment. Remember that survivorship is unique to each person, and there is no one-size-fits-all solution. Prioritize self-care, communicate openly with your healthcare team, and celebrate your progress. You are not alone, and there is help available as you navigate life after breast cancer treatment.

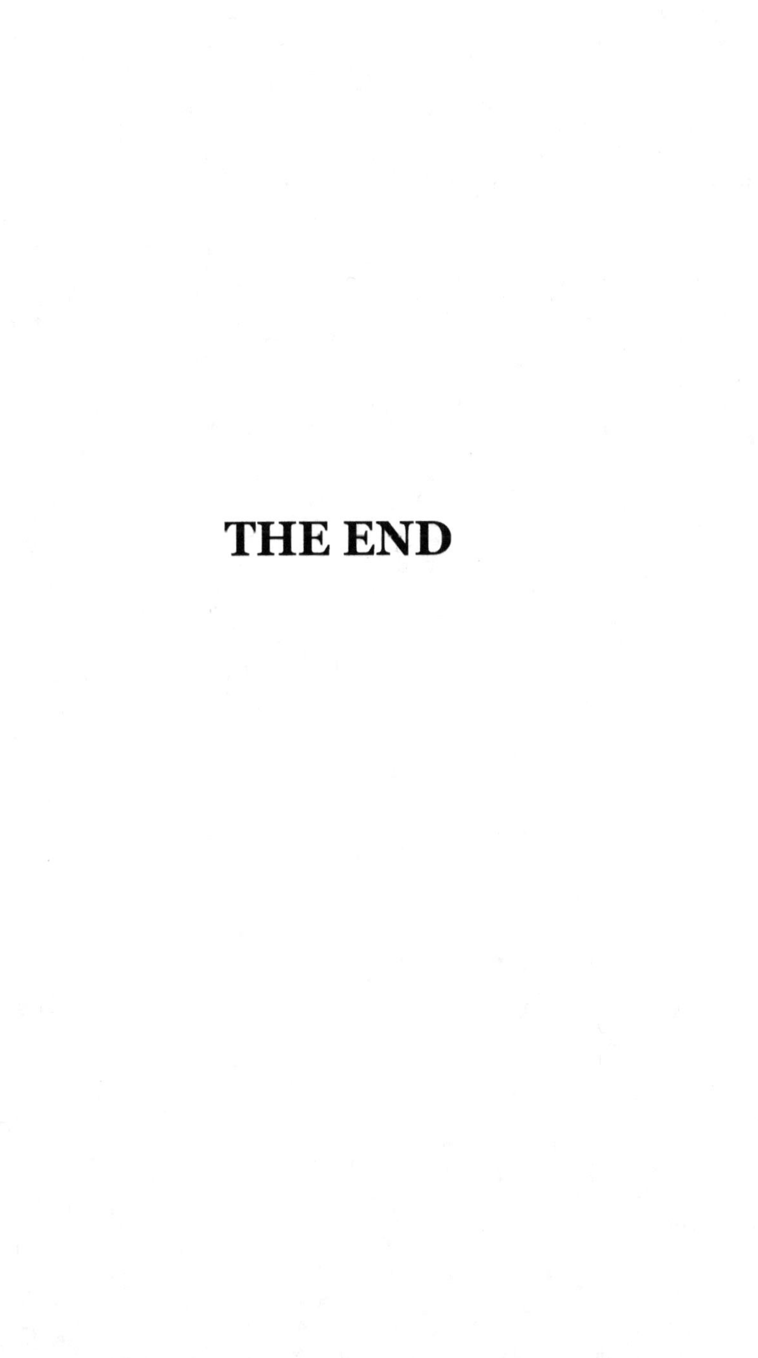

THE END

www.ingramcontent.com/pod-product-compliance
Lightning Source LLC
Chambersburg PA
CBHW070804250726
48662CB00004B/1962